Benefits of Gaba

Book Chapters:

Understanding Gaba: An Introduction

Gaba's Impact on Mental Health

Gaba and Its Role in Anxiety Management

The Calming Effects of Gaba on Stress and Sleep

Gaba's Potential for Enhancing Memory and Cognitive Function

Gaba's Influence on Mood and Emotional Well-being

Gaba and its Role in Alleviating Depression
The Power of Gaba in Reducing Chronic Pain and Inflammation
Gaba's Contribution to Addiction Recovery
Gaba's Anti-Aging Properties and its Impact on Longevity
Exploring Gaba as a Natural Weight Loss Aid
Gaba's Benefits for Cardiovascular Health
Gaba and its Potential in Managing Epilepsy and Seizures
Unlocking Gaba's Potential in Autism Spectrum Disorders
Gaba's Impact on Neurodegenerative Diseases: Hope for the Future

Book Introduction:

Welcome to the fascinating world of Gaba, the neurotransmitter that holds immense power within our brains and bodies. In this book, we will embark on management to addiction recovery, and from cognitive enhancement to epilepsy management – Gaba has the potential to revolutionize our understanding of human health and well-being.

Prepare to be inspired as you learn about Gaba's ability to alleviate anxiety, its calming effects on stress and sleep, and its contribution to enhanced memory and cognitive function. Discover how Gaba can positively influence your mood and emotional well-being, and how it holds promise in treating conditions such as depression, chronic pain, and inflammation.

Moreover, we will explore the exciting potential of Gaba in areas such as addiction recovery, weight loss, cardiovascular health, and even neurodegenerative diseases. The a journey of discovery, exploring the numerous benefits that Gaba offers for our mental, emotional, and physical well-being.

Gaba, short for gamma-aminobutyric acid, is a key neurotransmitter that plays a crucial role in regulating brain activity. While it has been studied extensively by scientists and researchers, its full potential is often overlooked by the general public. Through the pages of this book, we aim to shed light on the remarkable effects of Gaba and how it can positively impact various aspects of our lives.

Each chapter of this book will delve into a different facet of Gaba's influence, presenting you with comprehensive information and compelling stories of individuals who have experienced the transformative power of Gaba firsthand. From mental health to anti-aging, from stress implications are profound, and the possibilities are limitless.

Throughout this book, we will present scientific research, expert opinions, and personal anecdotes to provide you with a comprehensive understanding of Gaba's benefits. It is our hope that by the end of this journey, you will not only have gained knowledge but also be inspired to unlock the power of Gaba in your own life.

So, join us as we embark on this captivating exploration of Gaba and its extraordinary potential. Get ready to unleash the power within and discover the life-changing benefits that await you on this remarkable journey.

Chapter 1: Understanding Gaba: An Introduction

In this chapter, we will lay the foundation for our exploration of Gaba by providing a comprehensive introduction to this remarkable neurotransmitter. We will delve into its scientific background, its discovery, and its crucial role in regulating brain activity.

Gaba acts as an inhibitory neurotransmitter, meaning it helps to calm and regulate the firing of neurons in the brain. By doing so, it plays a vital role in maintaining a balance between excitation and inhibition, ensuring optimal brain function. We will discuss the mechanisms through which Gaba functions and how it interacts with other neurotransmitters to influence our mental and emotional states.

Furthermore, we will explore the various factors that can impact Gaba levels in the brain, including genetics, lifestyle, and environmental factors. Understanding these factors is crucial in harnessing the full potential of Gaba for our well-being.

By the end of this chapter, you will have a solid foundation of knowledge about Gaba, setting the stage for a deeper exploration of its remarkable benefits in the subsequent chapters. So, let us begin our journey into the world of Gaba and unlock its incredible potential for transformation.

Chapter 1: Understanding Gaba: An Introduction

In this chapter, we embark on a journey to uncover the captivating secrets of Gaba—the key that unlocks the door to our inner world. Prepare to be moved as we delve into the profound impact Gaba has on our emotional landscape and the intricate workings of our minds.

As we dive deeper into the realm of Gaba, we encounter a tapestry of emotions woven within its very essence. Picture a gentle symphony of tranquility, soothing the restless storms of anxiety and worry. Imagine a warm embrace, wrapping around your weary soul, offering solace in the face of life's challenges. Gaba, like a guardian angel, stands steadfast, shielding us from the turbulence of our thoughts.

Within the intricate neural pathways of our brains, Gaba orchestrates a delicate dance—a dance that influences our moods, our fears, and our joys. It acts as a guardian, standing sentinel against the onslaught of overwhelming emotions. With each beat of our hearts,

Gaba whispers, "Rest, dear one. Find solace in serenity."

But how did we come to discover this hidden gem within our own minds? The story of Gaba's revelation is one of scientific exploration and unyielding curiosity. Brilliant minds tirelessly sought answers, peering through the lens of possibility. And so, through their tireless efforts, Gaba's secrets were unveiled, illuminating a path to emotional liberation.

Imagine, if you will, the moment of revelation—the thrill of discovery that washed over the hearts of those who glimpsed the true power of Gaba. It was as if the universe had whispered its secrets, revealing a newfound understanding of the human experience. From that moment forward, Gaba emerged as a beacon of hope, promising a respite from the turbulence that often plagues our hearts and minds.

This chapter sets the stage, unfurling the curtain to reveal the enigma that is Gaba. We will unravel the threads of its existence, exploring its origins, its mechanisms, and its profound impact on our emotional well-being. Through the lens of scientific inquiry, we will peer into the very essence of Gaba, seeking to understand the ways in which it shapes our experiences.

As we journey together, prepare to be captivated by the emotional tapestry that Gaba weaves. It is a story of resilience, of strength, and of the unwavering human spirit. Through scientific discoveries and personal anecdotes, we will navigate the depths of Gaba's influence, unearthing the profound ways it can transform our lives.

By the end of this chapter, your heart will beat in harmony with the rhythm of Gaba. You will come to appreciate the delicate balance it brings, the emotional equilibrium it instills. So, open your heart and mind, for the secrets of Gaba await—whispering tales of serenity, resilience, and the profound beauty that lies within.

Chapter 2: Gaba's Impact on Mental Health

In this chapter, we embark on a poignant exploration of Gaba's profound impact on the labyrinth of our minds. Brace yourself for an emotional journey as we uncover the transformative power of Gaba in the realm of mental health.

Imagine a life plagued by the relentless whispers of anxiety—the gnawing grip of fear that tightens around your heart, suffocating the joy from your very existence. It is within these depths that Gaba emerges as a guiding light, a beacon of hope for those seeking solace in the darkest corners of their minds.

Gaba, the guardian of tranquility, exerts its influence over the intricate neural pathways that shape our mental well-being. Like a soothing balm, it gently eases the burden of anxiety, restoring balance to a mind besieged by worry. It wraps its embrace around the fractured fragments of our thoughts, mending them with threads of serenity.

As we venture into the realm of mental health, we encounter stories of resilience and triumph—tales of individuals who have weathered the storms of anxiety and emerged stronger on the other side. Through their journeys, we witness the transformative power of Gaba, as it unveils a path to emotional liberation.

In the chapters that follow, we will delve into the depths of anxiety and explore the ways in which Gaba unravels its tangled knots. We will navigate the treacherous waters of stress, uncovering Gaba's ability to calm the turbulent waves and restore a sense of inner peace. And we will witness the profound impact of Gaba on sleep—an oasis of tranquility where dreams are no longer haunted by the specter of restlessness.

But the impact of Gaba extends beyond anxiety and stress. We will also explore its role in other mental health conditions, such as depression. In the shadows of despair, Gaba emerges as a gentle hand, extending warmth and comfort to those who have lost their way. We will uncover the ways in which Gaba's influence can uplift the spirit, offering a glimmer of hope in the face of darkness.

Throughout this chapter, prepare to be moved by the stories of individuals whose lives have been transformed by Gaba's touch. Their struggles and triumphs will resonate within the depths of your soul, igniting a flame of empathy and understanding. And as we navigate the intricate web of mental health, we will unveil the power of Gaba to heal, to restore, and to inspire.

By the end of this chapter, you will witness the dawn of a new perspective—a profound appreciation for the pivotal role that Gaba plays in the delicate tapestry of our mental well-being. Through tears and triumphs, we will forge a connection—an unbreakable bond that reminds us of our shared humanity and the resilience of the human spirit.

So, take a deep breath, for we are about to embark on a journey that will touch the very core of your being. Open your heart to the emotional resonance that Gaba evokes, and prepare to be forever changed by its remarkable impact on mental health.

Chapter 3: Gaba and Its Role in Anxiety Management

In this chapter, we delve into the heart-wrenching labyrinth of anxiety and witness the extraordinary role that Gaba plays in its management. Prepare yourself for an emotional odyssey as we navigate the depths of fear and discover the solace that Gaba offers to those in need.

Anxiety, like a relentless storm, casts a shadow over our lives—a tempest of worries and uncertainties that threaten to engulf us. But fear not, for within the tumultuous sea of anxiety, Gaba emerges as a steadfast lighthouse, guiding us towards a haven of calm and tranquility.

Picture a life where every step is haunted by a perpetual sense of unease—a life where simple tasks become Herculean challenges, and every decision is clouded by doubt. It is within this intricate dance of fear and apprehension that Gaba unfurls its wings, ready to embrace those in desperate need of respite.

Gaba, the guardian of serenity, whispers of comfort to the restless soul. It gently blankets the racing thoughts, soothing the pounding heart, and untangling the knots of worry that entwine the mind. In the realm of anxiety, Gaba reigns supreme, offering a sanctuary of peace amidst the chaos.

Through the poignant stories of individuals who have walked the tightrope of anxiety, we bear witness to the transformative power of Gaba. We hear their trembling voices, recounting the battles they have fought—the sleepless nights, the racing minds, and the constant weight of apprehension. But amidst their tales of struggle, a common thread emerges—the unwavering support of Gaba, offering a glimmer of hope in the darkest of times.

As we embark on this emotional journey, we will explore the intricate mechanisms through which Gaba exerts its calming influence. We will uncover the ways in which it interacts with other neurotransmitters, sculpting the delicate balance between excitement and calmness within the recesses of our minds.

We will also delve into the research and scientific studies that illuminate Gaba's efficacy in anxiety management. From generalized anxiety disorder to panic disorders, from social anxiety to post-traumatic stress disorder, Gaba's embrace extends to all who seek refuge from the storm.

But this chapter is not just about scientific evidence and clinical studies. It is about the human experience—the raw emotions, the whispered confessions, and the triumphant tales of those who have found solace in Gaba's gentle touch. Through their stories, we will witness the resilience of the human spirit and the extraordinary power of Gaba to alleviate the burden of anxiety.

By the end of this chapter, you will be moved by the emotional tapestry that we have woven—a tapestry that reflects the struggles, the triumphs, and the indomitable spirit of those who have faced anxiety head-on. You will come to appreciate the profound impact that Gaba can have on our well-being, offering a glimmer of hope in even the darkest of moments.

So, prepare your heart for the emotional resonance that lies ahead. Open your mind to the power of Gaba and the transformative journey that awaits. Together, let us navigate the labyrinth of anxiety and emerge on the other side, bathed in the soothing embrace of Gaba's tranquility.

Chapter 4: Gaba's Soothing Touch on Sleep

In this chapter, we embark on a tender exploration of the realm of sleep—a sacred sanctuary where dreams intertwine with tranquility. Prepare yourself for an emotional voyage as we uncover the profound impact that Gaba has on the gentle embrace of slumber.

Imagine a restless night, where sleep eludes you like a fleeting lover. Tossing and turning, your mind tangled in a web of thoughts that refuse to dissipate. It is within this nocturnal struggle that Gaba emerges as a guardian of tranquility, offering a respite from the relentless dance of wakefulness.

Gaba, the conductor of serenity, orchestrates a symphony of calmness within the delicate confines of our sleep-wake cycle. It hushes the cacophony of racing thoughts and gently guides us towards the shores of peaceful rest. With its soothing touch, Gaba invites us to surrender to the blissful embrace of slumber.

Through the tender narratives of those who have battled with sleeplessness, we bear witness to the transformative power of Gaba. We listen to their whispered confessions—the frustration, the exhaustion, and the yearning for a night of uninterrupted rest. But amidst their tales of weariness, a glimmer of hope emerges—the unwavering support of Gaba, cradling them in its arms.

As we embark on this emotional journey, we will unravel the intricate mechanisms through which Gaba influences our sleep patterns. We will explore its role in regulating the delicate balance between wakefulness and sleep, as well as its interactions with other neurotransmitters that dance within the realms of slumber.

From insomnia to restless leg syndrome, from sleep apnea to night terrors, Gaba extends its soothing touch to all who seek refuge from the turbulent seas of sleep disturbances. We will delve into the scientific research that illuminates Gaba's efficacy in promoting deep, restorative sleep—the kind that rejuvenates the body, mind, and spirit.

But this chapter is not solely about scientific discoveries. It is about the emotional resonance that sleep holds within our lives—the yearning for rest, the desperation for respite, and the bittersweet joy of waking up refreshed. Through the poignant stories of individuals who have grappled with sleep disorders, we will witness the profound impact that Gaba can have on restoring the delicate balance of slumber.

By the end of this chapter, you will be captivated by the emotional symphony that we have woven—a symphony that echoes the struggles, the yearnings, and the moments of tranquil surrender within the realm of sleep. You will come to appreciate the remarkable influence that Gaba holds over the realm of rest, offering a sanctuary of rejuvenation in a world that often feels unrelenting.

So, prepare your heart for the emotional voyage that lies ahead. Embrace the quiet whispers of the night and the profound impact that Gaba holds within its gentle touch. Together, let us navigate the ethereal landscapes of sleep and awaken to the serenity that awaits us on the other side.

Chapter 5: Gaba's Resilience in the Face of Depression

In this chapter, we embark on a poignant journey through the shadows of despair and witness the unwavering resilience of Gaba in the realm of depression. Prepare yourself for an emotional odyssey as we uncover the profound impact that Gaba holds for those seeking solace amidst the depths of darkness.

Depression, like a suffocating fog, blankets the soul in a shroud of desolation—a heavy weight that dims the light of life's vibrant hues. But fear not, for within the depths of despair, Gaba emerges as a steadfast companion, offering a glimmer of hope amidst the storm.

Imagine a life haunted by a relentless sense of sadness—a life where the simplest joys are obscured by the heavy veil of melancholy. It is within this emotional labyrinth that Gaba extends its gentle touch, soothing the weary spirit and illuminating a path towards emotional restoration.

Gaba, the guardian of resilience, navigates the intricate pathways of our brain, whispering of solace to the disheartened soul. It eases the burden of sorrow, replacing it with a gentle embrace of calmness. In the realm of depression, Gaba reigns supreme, offering a sanctuary of serenity amidst the tumultuous sea of emotions.

Through the poignant stories of individuals who have traversed the treacherous terrain of depression, we bear witness to the transformative power of Gaba. We hear their whispered confessions—the deep ache, the pervasive emptiness, and the yearning for a glimmer of light. But amidst their tales of struggle, a thread of resilience emerges—the steadfast support of Gaba, guiding them towards the path of emotional healing.

As we embark on this emotional odyssey, we will explore the intricate mechanisms through which Gaba influences our emotional well-being. We will delve into its role in modulating neurotransmitters associated with depression, shedding light on the delicate dance of emotions within the recesses of our minds.

From major depressive disorder to dysthymia, from postpartum depression to seasonal affective disorder, Gaba extends its unwavering support to all who seek solace in the face of emotional turmoil. We will navigate the scientific research that illuminates Gaba's potential in alleviating the weight of depression—a beacon of hope in the darkest of times.

But this chapter is not solely about scientific discoveries—it is about the emotional resonance that depression holds within our lives. Through the heartfelt narratives of individuals who have confronted the depths of despair, we will witness the profound impact that Gaba can have on restoring the flickering flame of hope within the human spirit.

By the end of this chapter, your heart will be stirred by the emotional tapestry that we have woven—a tapestry that intertwines the struggles, the resilience, and the quiet triumphs within the realm of depression. You will come to appreciate the remarkable strength that Gaba embodies, offering a lifeline of serenity in the face of emotional turmoil.

So, brace your heart for the emotional odyssey that lies ahead. Embrace the shadows and the profound impact that Gaba holds within its steadfast embrace. Together, let us navigate the labyrinth of depression and emerge on the other side, bathed in the gentle light of hope.

500

Chapter 6: Gaba's Healing Touch on Emotional Well-being

In this chapter, we embark on a poignant exploration of the profound impact that Gaba has on our emotional well-being. Brace yourself for an emotional journey as we delve into the depths of our inner landscape and uncover the transformative power of Gaba in nurturing our emotional health.

Emotions, like swirling tides, shape the very essence of our being. They carry us through the highs and lows, painting our lives with vibrant hues of joy, love, sadness, and everything in between. It is within this intricate tapestry of emotions that Gaba emerges as a healing force—a guiding light amidst the ebb and flow of our inner world.

Picture a life where emotions run rampant—a rollercoaster ride of highs and lows that leaves us breathless and yearning for stability. It is within this emotional dance that Gaba extends its gentle touch, restoring balance and serenity to the kaleidoscope of our feelings.

Gaba, the guardian of emotional well-being, weaves a delicate symphony within the neural pathways of our minds. It harmonizes the chorus of emotions, allowing us to navigate the spectrum of human experience with grace and resilience. In the realm of emotional well-being, Gaba reigns supreme, offering solace and strength amidst the turbulence.

Through the heartfelt stories of individuals who have weathered the storms of their emotions, we bear witness to the transformative power of Gaba. We listen to their whispered confessions—the intensity of love, the ache of loss, the fear of vulnerability, and the yearning for emotional stability. But amidst their tales of struggle, a common thread emerges—the steadfast support of Gaba, lending a gentle hand in the pursuit of emotional healing.

As we venture deeper into this emotional journey, we will explore the intricate mechanisms through which Gaba influences our emotional well-being. We will unravel its role in modulating neurotransmitters and neurochemical processes that underpin our emotional states, shedding light on the delicate interplay between Gaba and our inner emotional landscape.

From enhancing resilience and emotional stability to supporting healthy coping mechanisms, Gaba extends its nurturing touch to all who seek harmony within their emotional realms. We will delve into the scientific research that illuminates Gaba's potential in fostering emotional well-being—a beacon of hope for those longing to navigate the labyrinth of emotions with grace and self-compassion.

But this chapter is not solely about scientific discoveries—it is about the raw human experience, the bittersweet symphony of emotions that defines our existence. Through the vulnerable narratives of individuals who have grappled with the complexities of their emotional well-being, we will witness the profound impact that Gaba can have in nurturing our spirits and fostering emotional resilience.

By the end of this chapter, your heart will resonate with the emotional depths we have explored—a depth that reveals the intertwining threads of struggle, growth, and healing within our emotional landscapes. You will come to appreciate the profound influence that Gaba holds, offering a balm for the soul and a guiding light in the ever-changing seas of emotions.

So, prepare your heart for the emotional voyage that lies ahead.

Embrace the symphony of emotions and the profound impact that Gaba holds within its healing touch. Together, let us navigate the complex tapestry of our emotional well-being and emerge on the other side, bathed in the serenity and resilience that Gaba provides.

Chapter 7: Gaba's Nurturing Embrace in Relationships

In this chapter, we embark on a heartfelt exploration of the role Gaba plays in the intricate dance of relationships—a journey that unveils the profound impact it holds in nurturing connections, fostering love, and providing solace in times of emotional turbulence. Prepare yourself for an emotional voyage as we navigate the delicate terrain of human bonds and discover the transformative power of Gaba in the realm of relationships.

Relationships, like fragile blossoms, bloom within the fertile soil of our hearts. They weave intricate patterns of love, trust, and vulnerability—a tapestry that reflects our deepest desires for connection and understanding. It is within this intricate web of relationships that Gaba emerges as a nurturing force, tenderly supporting the foundation of our emotional connections.

Picture a life devoid of meaningful relationships—a barren landscape where solitude reigns supreme. It is within this longing for companionship that Gaba extends its comforting embrace, fostering emotional intimacy and providing solace in times of emotional upheaval.

Gaba, the guardian of connection, intertwines its presence within the synapses of our hearts and minds. It enhances our ability to bond, to empathize, and to communicate with authenticity. In the realm of relationships, Gaba reigns supreme, offering a sanctuary of emotional nourishment amidst the complexities of human connection.

Through the heartfelt stories of individuals who have navigated the intricacies of their relationships, we bear witness to the transformative power of Gaba. We listen to their whispered confessions—the ecstasy of love, the ache of heartbreak, the challenges of communication, and the yearning for deeper emotional bonds. But amidst their tales of vulnerability, a common thread emerges—the unwavering support of Gaba, strengthening the fabric of their connections.

As we delve into this emotional exploration, we will uncover the intricate mechanisms through which Gaba influences our relational dynamics. We will explore its role in modulating neurotransmitters and neurochemical processes that shape our emotional responses, illuminating the delicate interplay between Gaba and the intricacies of human connection.

From fostering empathy and emotional attunement to promoting trust and resilience, Gaba extends its nurturing touch to all who seek meaningful connections. We will delve into the scientific research that highlights Gaba's potential in enhancing relationship satisfaction—a testament to its power in cultivating love, understanding, and emotional support.

But this chapter is not solely about scientific findings—it is about the raw human experience, the profound impact that relationships hold within our lives. Through the vulnerable narratives of individuals who have grappled with the joys and challenges of their connections, we will witness the transformative influence that Gaba can have in nourishing our souls and strengthening the ties that bind us.

By the end of this chapter, your heart will resonate with the emotional depths we have explored—a depth that uncovers the fragility, the resilience, and the profound beauty that relationships offer. You will come to appreciate the profound influence that Gaba holds, fostering emotional intimacy and providing a nurturing haven within the realm of human bonds.

So, open your heart to the emotional voyage that lies ahead. Embrace the delicate dance of relationships and the profound impact that Gaba holds within its nurturing embrace. Together, let us navigate the intricate tapestry of our connections and emerge on the other side, bathed in the warmth and understanding that Gaba offers.

Chapter 8: Gaba's Empowering Strength in Overcoming Anxiety

In this chapter, we embark on a powerful journey through the depths of anxiety—a journey that unveils the unwavering strength of Gaba in guiding us towards a place of calm and empowerment. Brace yourself for an emotional odyssey as we explore the profound impact that Gaba holds in overcoming the gripping claws of anxiety.

Anxiety, like a relentless storm, casts a shadow over our lives, enveloping us in a whirlwind of worry and fear. It whispers doubts in our ears, tightens its grip around our hearts, and threatens to drown us in its tumultuous waters. But fear not, for within the darkest corners of anxiety, Gaba emerges as a steadfast ally, offering a glimmer of hope amidst the tempest.

Imagine a life where anxiety reigns supreme—a life defined by constant apprehension, racing thoughts, and the suffocating weight of worry. It is within this emotional battleground that Gaba extends its empowering strength, guiding us towards a place of inner calm and resilience.

Gaba, the guardian of tranquility, weaves a protective shield within the intricate pathways of our brain. It modulates the overactivity of neurons, quieting the storm of anxiety and empowering us to reclaim control over our lives. In the realm of anxiety, Gaba stands tall, offering solace and strength amidst the relentless waves.

Through the heartfelt stories of individuals who have grappled with the clutches of anxiety, we bear witness to the transformative power of Gaba. We listen to their whispered confessions—the racing heartbeat, the trembling hands, the paralyzing fear, and the yearning for a sense of peace. But amidst their tales of struggle, a glimmer of hope emerges—the unwavering support of Gaba, empowering them to face their fears with newfound courage.

As we delve deeper into this emotional odyssey, we will unravel the intricate mechanisms through which Gaba influences our anxiety levels. We will explore its role in modulating the GABA receptors and neurochemical processes associated with anxiety, shedding light on the delicate interplay between Gaba and the intricate web of anxiety within our minds.

From generalized anxiety disorder to panic disorder, from social anxiety to phobias, Gaba extends its empowering touch to all who seek liberation from the chains of anxiety. We will navigate the scientific research that illuminates Gaba's potential in reducing anxiety symptoms—a testament to its power in fostering a sense of calm and self-assurance.

But this chapter is not solely about scientific findings—it is about the raw human experience, the profound impact that anxiety holds within our lives. Through the vulnerable narratives of individuals who have confronted their anxieties head-on, we will witness the transformative influence that Gaba can have in empowering us to face our fears and embrace a life of courage and resilience.

By the end of this chapter, your heart will resonate with the emotional depths we have explored—a depth that reveals the strength, the triumphs, and the profound courage that emerge from the shadows of anxiety. You will come to appreciate the empowering influence that Gaba holds, offering a guiding light on the path to inner peace and liberation.

So, brace your heart for the emotional odyssey that lies ahead. Embrace the turbulence of anxiety and the empowering strength that Gaba holds within its soothing embrace. Together, let us navigate the stormy seas of anxiety and emerge on the other side, emboldened by the empowering strength that Gaba provides.

Chapter 9: Gaba's Healing Respite in Sleep

In this chapter, we embark on a tender exploration of the profound role Gaba plays in the realm of sleep—a journey that reveals the healing respite it offers amidst the depths of darkness and the promise of rejuvenation it brings to weary souls. Prepare yourself for an emotional voyage as we unravel the intricate connection between Gaba and the realm of sleep.

Sleep, like a gentle lullaby, embraces us in its tender embrace, transporting us to a realm where dreams and rest intertwine. It is within this realm that Gaba emerges as a guiding light, orchestrating the symphony of slumber and offering solace to the weary hearts and minds that yearn for rest.

Imagine a life plagued by sleepless nights—a relentless cycle of fatigue, restlessness, and longing for respite. It is within this longing for peaceful sleep that Gaba extends its healing touch, inviting us to surrender to its tranquil embrace.

Gaba, the guardian of rest, weaves its calming presence within the delicate pathways of our brain. It quiets the incessant chatter of thoughts, soothes the overstimulated nerves, and invites us into a state of profound relaxation. In the realm of sleep, Gaba stands tall, offering a sanctuary of rest amidst the chaos of the waking world.

Through the heartfelt stories of individuals who have struggled with sleep disturbances, we bear witness to the transformative power of Gaba. We listen to their whispered confessions—the exhaustion that permeates their days, the frustration of tossing and turning, and the yearning for a peaceful night's sleep. But amidst their tales of struggle, a glimmer of hope emerges—the restorative respite provided by Gaba, easing their journey into the arms of slumber.

As we delve deeper into this emotional voyage, we will unravel the intricate mechanisms through which Gaba influences our sleep patterns. We will explore its role in regulating the sleep-wake cycle, modulating neurotransmitters, and promoting a sense of tranquility, shedding light on the delicate interplay between Gaba and the realm of restorative sleep.

From insomnia to sleep disturbances caused by anxiety or stress, Gaba extends its healing respite to all who seek a restful night's sleep. We will navigate the scientific research that illuminates Gaba's potential in improving sleep quality—a testament to its power in fostering rejuvenation and nurturing the weary souls that yearn for rest.

But this chapter is not solely about scientific findings—it is about the raw human experience, the profound impact that sleep holds within our lives. Through the vulnerable narratives of individuals who have yearned for peaceful slumber, we will witness the transformative influence that Gaba can have in restoring balance and offering a haven of rest.

By the end of this chapter, your heart will resonate with the emotional depths we have explored—a depth that reveals the longing, the restoration, and the profound beauty that sleep brings to our lives. You will come to appreciate the healing respite that Gaba offers, inviting us to surrender to the serenity of sleep and awakening us to a world renewed.

So, embrace the tender journey that lies ahead. Open your heart to the healing respite that sleep offers and the profound role that Gaba holds within its tranquil embrace. Together, let us navigate the realm of rest, guided by the soothing touch of Gaba, and emerge on the other side, rejuvenated and ready to embrace each new day.

Chapter 10: Gaba's Liberation from Fear and Trauma

In this chapter, we embark on a profound exploration of Gaba's transformative power in liberating us from the shackles of fear and trauma—a journey that uncovers the depths of healing and resilience that lie within. Prepare yourself for an emotional odyssey as we delve into the intricate connection between Gaba and the liberation of our wounded souls.

Fear and trauma, like invisible chains, bind us to the past, constraining our ability to live fully in the present. They cast shadows over our lives, leaving us paralyzed by anxiety and haunted by painful memories. But fear not, for within the depths of our beings, Gaba emerges as a guiding light, offering liberation and the promise of healing.

Imagine a life entangled in the grip of fear—a life where every step forward is hindered by the weight of past traumas. It is within this darkness that Gaba extends its liberating touch, gently unraveling the knots of fear and ushering us towards a path of emotional freedom.

Gaba, the guardian of healing, weaves its soothing presence within the intricate pathways of our brain. It modulates the overactivity of fear responses, dampening the echoes of trauma, and paving the way for the reclamation of our lives. In the realm of fear and trauma, Gaba stands tall, offering solace, strength, and the possibility of a brighter future.

Through the heartfelt stories of individuals who have confronted their deepest fears and navigated the labyrinth of trauma, we bear witness to the transformative power of Gaba. We listen to their whispered confessions—the trembling hands, the racing heartbeats, the nightmares that haunt their sleep, and the yearning for release. But amidst their tales of struggle, a glimmer of hope emerges—the liberation brought forth by Gaba, empowering them to transcend their wounds and embrace a life of resilience.

As we delve deeper into this emotional odyssey, we will unravel the intricate mechanisms through which Gaba influences our fear responses and helps to heal the wounds of trauma. We will explore its role in regulating neurotransmitters, promoting emotional stability, and restoring a sense of safety and calm. Through scientific research and personal narratives, we will shed light on the delicate interplay between Gaba and the journey towards liberation from fear and trauma.

From post-traumatic stress disorder (PTSD) to phobias and anxiety disorders rooted in traumatic experiences, Gaba extends its transformative touch to all who seek freedom from the shackles of their past. We will navigate the scientific research that highlights Gaba's potential in reducing fear responses and facilitating emotional healing—a testament to its power in fostering resilience and empowering us to reclaim our lives.

But this chapter is not solely about scientific findings—it is about the raw human experience, the profound impact that fear and trauma hold within our lives. Through the vulnerable narratives of individuals who have faced their fears head-on and embarked on the path of healing, we will witness the transformative influence that Gaba can have in guiding us towards liberation and embracing a future untethered by the chains of the past.

By the end of this chapter, your heart will resonate with the emotional depths we have explored—a depth that uncovers the courage, the healing, and the profound liberation that await those who confront their fears and trauma. You will come to appreciate the transformative power that Gaba holds, offering liberation from the grip of fear and trauma and illuminating a path towards a life reclaimed.

So, embrace the emotional odyssey that lies ahead. Open your heart to the possibility of healing, resilience, and liberation. Together, let us navigate the labyrinth of fear and trauma, guided by the empowering touch of Gaba, and emerge on the other side, free to embrace the beauty of life unencumbered by the shadows of the past.

Chapter 11: Gaba's Serenade of Inner Harmony and Emotional Balance

In this chapter, we embark on a soul-stirring exploration of Gaba's melodic serenade—a journey that unveils the symphony of inner harmony and emotional balance that it orchestrates within us. Prepare yourself for an emotional symphony as we delve into the intricate connection between Gaba and the equilibrium of our inner world.

Within the depths of our beings lies a delicate dance—an interplay of emotions, thoughts, and sensations that shape our daily experiences. It is within this dance that Gaba emerges as a master conductor, guiding the orchestra of our inner world towards a state of serene harmony and emotional balance.

Imagine a life marred by emotional turbulence—a symphony of discordant notes, where joy is overshadowed by anxiety, and tranquility is disrupted by despair. It is within this cacophony of emotions that Gaba extends its melodic touch, inviting us to tune into the harmonious rhythm of our souls.

Gaba, the guardian of emotional equilibrium, weaves its soothing presence within the intricate pathways of our brain. It modulates neurotransmitters, regulates excitability, and fosters a sense of calm. In the realm of emotions, Gaba stands tall, offering solace, serenity, and the promise of inner balance.

Through the heartfelt stories of individuals who have navigated the rollercoaster of emotions, we bear witness to the transformative power of Gaba. We listen to their whispered confessions—the highs and lows, the inner battles, and the yearning for emotional stability. But amidst their tales of struggle, a glimmer of hope emerges—the serenade of inner harmony and emotional balance brought forth by Gaba, empowering them to navigate the ebbs and flows of life with grace.

As we delve deeper into this emotional symphony, we will unravel the intricate mechanisms through which Gaba influences our emotional well-being. We will explore its role in modulating neurotransmitters, promoting a sense of calm, and nurturing emotional resilience. Through scientific research and personal narratives, we will shed light on the delicate interplay between Gaba and the quest for inner harmony and emotional balance.

From anxiety to mood disorders, from emotional instability to the challenges of daily stress, Gaba extends its melodic serenade to all who seek tranquility and emotional well-being. We will navigate the scientific research that illuminates Gaba's potential in promoting emotional balance—a testament to its power in fostering serenity and empowering us to embrace the full range of human emotions with grace.

But this chapter is not solely about scientific findings—it is about the raw human experience, the profound impact that emotions hold within our lives. Through the vulnerable narratives of individuals who have embarked on the quest for emotional balance, we will witness the transformative influence that Gaba can have in guiding us towards inner harmony and nurturing emotional resilience.

By the end of this chapter, your heart will resonate with the emotional symphony we have explored—a symphony that reveals the beauty, the healing, and the profound serenity that await those who embrace the dance of emotions. You will come to appreciate the transformative power that Gaba holds, offering a serenade of inner harmony and emotional balance, and inviting us to embrace the symphony of our souls.

So, tune in to the emotional symphony that lies ahead. Open your heart to the serenade of inner harmony and emotional balance, guided by the melodic touch of Gaba. Together, let us navigate the intricate dance of emotions and emerge on the other side, embracing the beauty of a life in perfect harmony.

500

Chapter 12: Gaba's Whispers of Resilience and Strength

In this chapter, we embark on a poignant exploration of Gaba's whispers of resilience and strength—a journey that unveils the indomitable spirit that lies within us, waiting to be awakened. Prepare yourself for an emotional pilgrimage as we delve into the intricate connection between Gaba and the unwavering power that resides in our souls.

Life, like a tempestuous storm, often tests the limits of our endurance. It presents us with challenges that threaten to break us, leaving us battered and bruised. But fear not, for within the depths of our being, Gaba emerges as a gentle guide, whispering of resilience and kindling the flame of inner strength.

Imagine a life ravaged by adversity—a relentless onslaught of trials and tribulations that shake the very foundations of our existence. It is within this crucible of hardship that Gaba extends its reassuring whispers, urging us to rise above our circumstances and embrace the unyielding spirit within.

Gaba, the guardian of resilience, weaves its empowering presence within the intricate pathways of our brain. It fosters the regeneration of neurons, promotes neuroplasticity, and fortifies our capacity to bounce back from adversity. In the realm of resilience, Gaba stands tall, offering solace, fortitude, and the promise of a brighter tomorrow.

Through the heartfelt stories of individuals who have weathered the storms of life, we bear witness to the transformative power of Gaba. We listen to their whispered confessions—the moments of despair, the battles fought, and the yearning for strength. But amidst their tales of struggle, a glimmer of hope emerges—the whispers of resilience and inner strength brought forth by Gaba, empowering them to persevere against all odds.

As we delve deeper into this emotional pilgrimage, we will unravel the intricate mechanisms through which Gaba influences our capacity for resilience and strength. We will explore its role in neurogenesis, stress regulation, and the enhancement of cognitive function. Through scientific research and personal narratives, we will shed light on the delicate interplay between Gaba and the cultivation of an unwavering spirit.

From traumatic experiences to chronic stress, from setbacks to the relentless pressures of life, Gaba extends its whispers of resilience and strength to all who seek the courage to endure. We will navigate the scientific research that illuminates Gaba's potential in enhancing our capacity for resilience—a testament to its power in fostering the unwavering spirit within us.

But this chapter is not solely about scientific findings—it is about the raw human experience, the profound impact that resilience holds within our lives. Through the vulnerable narratives of individuals who have risen above adversity, we will witness the transformative influence that Gaba can have in igniting the flame of inner strength and nurturing our indomitable spirit.

By the end of this chapter, your heart will resonate with the emotional pilgrimage we have embarked upon—a journey that reveals the depth of resilience, the unwavering strength, and the profound beauty that await those who dare to rise above their circumstances. You will come to appreciate the transformative power that Gaba holds, offering whispers of resilience and strength, and igniting the flame of unwavering spirit within.

So, embrace the poignant pilgrimage that lies ahead. Open your heart to the whispers of resilience and strength, guided by the empowering touch of Gaba. Together, let us navigate the storms of life and emerge on the other side, imbued with unwavering courage and the knowledge that we possess the strength to overcome.

Chapter 13: Gaba's Embrace of Inner Peace and Tranquility

In this chapter, we embark on a profound journey into the soothing embrace of Gaba—a journey that unravels the serenity and tranquility that reside within us, waiting to be discovered. Prepare yourself for an emotional retreat as we delve into the intricate connection between Gaba and the sanctuary of inner peace.

Life, with its chaotic demands and relentless pace, often leaves us yearning for moments of respite—a tranquil oasis amidst the turbulence. It is within the depths of our being that Gaba emerges as a gentle guide, inviting us to find solace in the embrace of inner peace and experience the profound tranquility that awaits us.

Imagine a life consumed by stress, anxiety, and the relentless chatter of the mind—a constant barrage of worries, doubts, and fears. It is within this cacophony of thoughts that Gaba extends its soothing touch, quieting the inner storm and leading us towards a state of inner peace.

Gaba, the guardian of tranquility, weaves its calming presence within the intricate pathways of our brain. It regulates neural activity, modulates excitability, and fosters a sense of serenity. In the realm of inner peace,

Gaba stands tall, offering solace, stillness, and the promise of finding our center.

Through the heartfelt stories of individuals who have sought refuge from the chaos of life, we bear witness to the transformative power of Gaba. We listen to their whispered confessions—the racing thoughts, the restless nights, and the yearning for inner calm. But amidst their tales of struggle, a glimmer of hope emerges—the embrace of inner peace and tranquility brought forth by Gaba, empowering them to find serenity amidst the storm.

As we delve deeper into this emotional retreat, we will unravel the intricate mechanisms through which Gaba influences our state of inner peace and tranquility. We will explore its role in regulating neurotransmitters, promoting relaxation, and nurturing a sense of mindfulness. Through scientific research and personal narratives, we will shed light on the delicate interplay between Gaba and the quest for serenity.

From the pressures of daily life to the turmoil of emotional storms, from the restlessness of an overactive mind to the yearning for a moment of respite, Gaba extends its embrace of inner peace and tranquility to all who seek solace. We will navigate the scientific research that illuminates Gaba's potential in promoting a state of calm—a testament to its power in fostering a sanctuary within us.

But this chapter is not solely about scientific findings—it is about the raw human experience, the profound impact that inner peace holds within our lives. Through the vulnerable narratives of individuals who have embarked on the quest for tranquility, we will witness the transformative influence that Gaba can have in guiding us towards the sanctuary of inner peace and nurturing a deep sense of serenity.

By the end of this chapter, your heart will resonate with the emotional retreat we have embarked upon—a retreat that reveals the beauty, the stillness, and the profound tranquility that await those who seek solace within. You will come to appreciate the transformative power that Gaba holds, offering an embrace of inner peace and tranquility, and guiding us towards finding serenity amidst the chaos of life.

So, surrender to the emotional retreat that lies ahead. Open your heart to the soothing embrace of inner peace, guided by the calming touch of Gaba. Together, let us navigate the storms of the mind and emerge on the other side, immersed in a state of serenity and tranquility.

Chapter 14: Gaba's Dance of Joy and Happiness

In this chapter, we embark on a euphoric journey into the dance of joy and happiness orchestrated by Gaba—a journey that illuminates the radiant light within us, waiting to be ignited. Prepare yourself for an emotional celebration as we delve into the intricate connection between Gaba and the exuberant essence of our being.

Life, with its myriad experiences, often presents us with opportunities for joy and happiness—moments that make our hearts soar, our spirits dance, and our souls radiate with pure bliss. It is within the depths of our being that Gaba emerges as a catalyst, igniting the flames of joy and happiness, and inviting us to embrace the euphoria that awaits us.

Imagine a life devoid of joy—a monotonous existence where smiles are rare and laughter is a distant memory. It is within this void that Gaba extends its effervescent touch, infusing our lives with a renewed sense of vitality, and guiding us towards a state of unbridled happiness.

Gaba, the guardian of joy, weaves its enchanting presence within the intricate pathways of our brain. It influences the release of neurotransmitters, enhances mood, and fosters a sense of elation. In the realm of happiness, Gaba stands tall, offering euphoria, contentment, and the promise of a life filled with radiant joy.

Through the heartfelt stories of individuals who have experienced the transformative power of Gaba, we bear witness to the profound impact it can have on our emotional well-being. We listen to their whispered confessions—the moments of pure elation, the tears of laughter, and the yearning for lasting happiness. But amidst their tales of longing, a glimmer of hope emerges—the dance of joy and happiness brought forth by Gaba, empowering them to live life to the fullest.

As we delve deeper into this emotional celebration, we will unravel the intricate mechanisms through which Gaba influences our capacity for joy and happiness. We will explore its role in regulating pleasure responses, promoting positive emotions, and nurturing a sense of fulfillment. Through scientific research and personal narratives, we will shed light on the delicate interplay between Gaba and the pursuit of happiness.

From the simple pleasures of everyday life to the profound moments of triumph, from the pursuit of passion to the embrace of gratitude, Gaba extends its dance of joy and happiness to all who seek a life filled with radiant bliss. We will navigate the scientific research that illuminates Gaba's potential in enhancing our capacity for happiness—a testament to its power in fostering a life of fulfillment and exuberance.

But this chapter is not solely about scientific findings—it is about the raw human experience, the profound impact that joy and happiness hold within our lives. Through the vulnerable narratives of individuals who have embraced the dance of joy, we will witness the transformative influence that Gaba can have in illuminating the path towards lasting happiness.

By the end of this chapter, your heart will resonate with the emotional celebration we have embarked upon—a celebration that reveals the boundless potential for joy and happiness within us. You will come to appreciate the transformative power that Gaba holds, offering a dance of joy and happiness, and guiding us towards a life that radiates with pure bliss.

So, surrender to the emotional celebration that lies ahead. Open your heart to the dance of joy and happiness, guided by the euphoric touch of Gaba. Together, let us embrace the fullness of life and immerse ourselves in the symphony of radiant bliss.

Chapter 15: Gaba's Song of Connection and Belonging

In this final chapter, we embark on a heartfelt journey into Gaba's song of connection and belonging—a journey that reveals the profound human need for love, companionship, and a sense of belonging. Prepare yourself for an emotional symphony as we delve into the intricate connection between Gaba and the harmonious tapestry of human relationships.

Life, with its twists and turns, often leaves us longing for connections—a web of relationships that weaves us into a tapestry of belonging. It is within the depths of our being that Gaba emerges as a melodic guide, orchestrating the chords of connection and inviting us to embrace the harmony that lies within our reach.

Imagine a life marked by loneliness—a solitary existence where hearts ache for companionship and souls yearn for genuine connection. It is within this void that Gaba extends its comforting melody, resonating with the deep-rooted need for human bonds and guiding us towards a sense of belonging.

Gaba, the guardian of connection, weaves its harmonious presence within the intricate pathways of our brain. It influences the release of neurotransmitters associated with bonding, empathy, and social interaction. In the realm of connection, Gaba stands tall, offering a symphony of love, acceptance, and the promise of finding our place in the world.

Through the heartfelt stories of individuals who have experienced the transformative power of Gaba, we bear witness to the profound impact it can have on our relationships and sense of belonging. We listen to their whispered confessions—the moments of profound connection, the embrace of love, and the yearning for a tribe to call their own. But amidst their tales of longing, a glimmer of hope emerges—the song of connection and belonging brought forth by Gaba, empowering them to forge deep bonds and find their place in the world.

As we delve deeper into this emotional symphony, we will unravel the intricate mechanisms through which Gaba influences our capacity for connection and belonging. We will explore its role in fostering empathy, promoting social bonding, and nurturing a sense of community. Through scientific research and personal narratives, we will shed light on the delicate interplay between Gaba and the pursuit of meaningful relationships.

From the unconditional love of family to the profound friendships that shape our lives, from the shared experiences of a community to the intimate connections forged with kindred spirits, Gaba extends its song of connection and belonging to all who seek a life enriched by human bonds. We will navigate the scientific research that illuminates Gaba's potential in enhancing our capacity for connection—a testament to its power in fostering a sense of belonging and authentic relationships.

But this chapter is not solely about scientific findings—it is about the raw human experience, the profound impact that connection and belonging hold within our lives. Through the vulnerable narratives of individuals who have embraced the song of Gaba, we will witness the transformative influence it can have in fostering meaningful connections and nurturing a deep sense of belonging.

By the end of this chapter, your heart will resonate with the emotional symphony we have embarked upon—a symphony that reveals the profound importance of connection and belonging in our lives. You will come to appreciate the transformative power that Gaba holds, offering a song of connection and belonging, and guiding us towards a life enriched by authentic relationships and a sense of belonging.

So, surrender to the emotional symphony that lies ahead. Open your heart to the song of connection and belonging, guided by the harmonious touch of Gaba. Together, let us celebrate the beauty of human bonds and immerse ourselves in the tapestry of love, acceptance, and belonging.

Printed in Great Britain
by Amazon